Intermittent Fasting

The Secret Weapon to Burning Fat and Building Muscle With Ease

Thomas Rohmer

Copyright © 2017

Rohmerfitness All rights reserved.

No part of this publication may be reproduced, distributed, or transmitted in any form or by any means, including photocopying, recording, or other electronic or mechanical methods, without the prior written permission and consent of the publisher, except in the in the case of brief quotations embodied in product reviews and certain other non-commercial uses permitted by copyright law.

Disclaimer:

This guide has been created for informational and reference purposes only. The author, publisher, and any other affiliated parties cannot be held in any way accountable for any personal injuries or damage allegedly resulting from the information contained herein, or from any misuse of such guidance. Although strict measures have been taken to provide accurate information, the parties involved with the creation and publication of this guide take no responsibility for any issues that many arise from alleged discrepancies contained herein. It is strongly recommended that you consult a physician, personal trainer, and nutritionist prior to commencing this or any other workout or diet plan. This guide is not a substitute for professional personal guidance from a qualified medical professional. If you feel pain or discomfort at any point during exercises contained herein, cease the activity immediately and seek medical guidance.

Table of Contents

Chapter 1: The Diet Trap You've Fallen Victim To...4

Chapter 2: What the Heck is a Calorie Anyway?......6

Chapter 3: History of Fasting...................................11

Chapter 4: Benefits of Fasting..................................14

Chapter 5: Different Methods of Fasting................16

Chapter 6: Fasting and Exercise..............................24

Chapter 7: Fasting and Building Muscle................28

Chapter 8: Muscle Building Workout With Fasting..34

Chapter 9: How You Can Actually Be Successful With Your Fitness Journey....................................36

Chapter 10: Frequently Asked Questions...............39

Chapter 1: The Diet Trap You've Fallen Victim To

Tell me if this story sounds familiar to you:

1. You want to lose weight.
2. You go on a diet.
3. You eliminate all junk food and eat healthy 24/7.
4. After a week, you start to get worn out.
5. You get tempted by a chocolate chip cookie and eat it.
6. You feel guilty and binge eat everything in sight.
7. A few days later, when you're feeling better about yourself, you start the process over again.

Of the 45 million Americans (1) who'll go on a diet this year, a story similar to this will be a reality for most of them.

1. Go on a diet.
2. Make yourself miserable.
3. Quit when you can't take it anymore and gain all of the weight back.

That's the problem with the word "diet." It suggests short-term change. When someone goes *on* a diet they must eventually go *off* a diet. When that happens, rebound weight gain will occur. Fortunately, there's a much better option out there than a typical "diet."

Why Fasting is Different

Dieting doesn't work because it isn't sustainable for the long haul. Seriously, do you really think you can eat chicken breast and salad for the rest of your life? You must do something different from the norm if you want to see lasting results. This is where fasting comes into play. Fasting is a great fat loss solution because you can easily do it for the rest of your life. You can fast to get lean, and then you can keep fasting to stay lean. No gimmicky diets, pills, or powders will ever be needed. Before we get into the ins and outs of fasting, it's first important to understand how your body works in regards to losing weight.

Chapter 2: What the Heck is a Calorie Anyway?

You've undoubtedly heard of the word calorie before. But what exactly is a calorie anyway? Is it something evil you should avoid whenever possible? Is it the bane of your existence?

Many people have an idea of what a calorie is, but most don't know. If you went out on the street and asked 10 different people what a calorie is, you'd likely get 10 different answers. Here's the textbook definition of a calorie:

"The energy needed to raise the temperature of 1 gram of water through 1° C"

Sounds complicated right? Essentially, a calorie is a measurement of energy. Your body is constantly undergoing chemical reactions to keep you alive. All of these chemical reactions (digestion, breathing, organ function, etc.) require energy.

Your body gets the energy necessary to continue functioning from the food (calories) you eat. Calories aren't your worst enemy; they're your friend. You have to work with them, not against them. And as you're about to find out, not all calories are the same.

Is a Calorie a Calorie?

This is a big debate in the fitness industry. If I eat 100 calories from a candy bar, and you eat 100 calories worth of vegetables, are we equal? Well, yes and no.

One calorie *is* one calorie regardless of what source the calorie came from. Trying to argue with this is like saying one yard going east isn't the same distance as going one yard west. The difference lies in the *macronutrient* quality.

100 calories from vegetables and 100 calories from candy is still 100 calories. Both are made up mostly of carbs; the quality of those carbs is what makes them very different. The candy contains simple carbs and sugar.

It won't provide you with any vitamins, nutrients, or fiber. It also won't be very satiating. The vegetables, on the other hand, are complex carbs.

They'll provide you with quality complex carbs and a good source of vitamins, nutrients, and fiber. Additionally, nutritious food like fruits and vegetables will keep you fuller longer, which is critical during calorie restriction for weight loss purposes. Therefore, quality of calories can be just as important as quantity of calories.

The Caloric Deficit is King

Pop quiz: What's the *only* way your body can burn fat?

If you looked at the title above and guessed caloric deficit, then you'd be correct! A caloric deficit is simply when you burn off more calories than you consume. The opposite is a caloric surplus—consuming more calories than you burn off. And maintenance is when you are at a caloric equilibrium.

Here's an example:

-Joe burns 2,000 calories a day and eats 1,800. He's in a caloric deficit of 200 calories and he'll start to lose weight.
-Joe burns 2,000 calories a day and eats 2,200. He's in a caloric surplus of 200 calories and he'll start to gain weight.
-Joe burns 2,000 calories a day and eats 2,000. He's at maintenance and will not gain or lose weight.

As I mentioned earlier, every day your body needs energy (calories) in order to continue on with all of its chemical functions such as breathing, digesting food, organ function, etc. The amount of calories you burn in any given day is your resting metabolic rate (rmr). Once you figure out your body's rmr, you can then determine how many calories you need to eat to start burning fat.

Determining your rmr is simple—multiply your bodyweight in pounds by 13.
Let's use myself as an example:

Bodyweight=195 pounds
195 x 13= RMR of 2,535

This means that if I eat less than 2,535 calories I'll be in a caloric deficit and I'll start to lose weight. If I eat more than 2,535 calories I'll be in a caloric surplus and I'll start to gain weight. And finally, if I eat exactly 2,535 calories, I'll be at maintenance and I'll neither gain nor lose weight.

The question is—how big of a caloric deficit do you need to create in order for it to translate into pounds lost? There's about 3,500 calories in one pound of fat (2), meaning that you must create a cumulative caloric deficit of 3,500 calories in order to lose 1 pound. So if you divide 3,500 by 7 days in a week, you'll need to create an average daily caloric deficit of 500 calories to lose 1 pound per week.

Referring back to the example from above, here's what that would translate to:

RMR- 2,535 – 500= 2,035

This means that I need to eat 2,035 calories everyday if I want to lose 1 pound per week. The more weight you have to lose, the larger the caloric deficit you can create. For example, you could eat at a caloric deficit of 750 calories and lose 1.5 pounds per week, or you could eat at a deficit of 1,000 calories to lose 2 pounds per week.
Essentially, for every 250 calories you can expect to lose an additional .5-pound. The key is to not get carried away. You

might want to lose all of the weight as soon as possible and jump right into a 1,000-calorie caloric deficit.

That may not be the best idea. For most people, losing 1 pound per week by creating a 500-calorie caloric deficit is golden. Imagine yourself a year from now being 52 pounds lighter without having to put forth much effort! That's much better than spinning your wheels trying to lose 100 pounds in that same time frame.

Here's a chart you can use to determine the rate you should lose weight at:

Amount of Weight You Need to Lose	Rate at Which You Should Lose Weight
≥5-10 pounds	.5 pound per week
10-30 pounds	1 pound per week
30+ pounds	1.5-2+ pounds per week

Here's the kicker:

What if you don't know how much weight you need to lose to look the way you want to? This is a good question because you won't know how much you need to weigh to look good until you reach that point. Therefore, you'll simply have to take your best guess as to what your goal weight is and adjust it once you reach it.

For example, let's say someone weighs 200 pounds. This individual could pick a goal weight of 180 pounds and start losing weight at a rate of 1 pound per week. Once he reaches his goal of 180 pounds, he can see if he's satisfied with how he looks.

If he's happy with how he looks, then great. If not, then he needs to readjust his goal. He could set his new target weight at 170 pounds and lose weight at a rate of .5 to 1 pound per week, continuing the process until he's happy with his leanness.

What is Fasting?

Intermittent fasting is simply taking a break from eating for a prolonged period of time. I'll get into the different styles of fasting that exist in a bit, but for now know this—when you fast, you don't eat. Every diet that has ever been created is designed to put you into a caloric deficit one way or another.

For example, a low-carb diet will reduce overall calories by reducing carb intake. Going on a diet consisting of nothing but healthy foods will try to achieve the same goal by eliminating high calorie junk food items. Fasting is no different, and its main way of getting you into a caloric deficit will be by reducing meal frequency.

Unlike low-carb or eating healthy 24/7, you'll actually be able to fast for a long time to come. Not only that, but it's also an enjoyable nutrition plan once you get used to it! Is giving up your favorite foods fun? Heck no! Luckily, fasting allows you to have your cake and eat it too.

Chapter 3: History of Fasting

Fasting isn't a new idea even though it has gained popularity in recent times. People have been fasting for thousands of years for various reasons—religious purposes, preparing for war, political protests, healing of illnesses (before medicine became prevalent), and even out of necessity. Muslims fast while the sun is up during the month of Ramadan.

Roman Catholics fast for 40 days during Lent to represent the 40 days Jesus fasted in the desert. Judaism has several annual fasts as well. Fasting was sometimes demanded before going to war as part of a ritual. And figures like Mahatma Gandhi have fasted for 21 days straight during the struggle for Indian independence.

It wasn't until recently that people began fasting for the enhanced health and fat loss benefits. Imagine for a second that you're a nomadic hunter and gather living thousands of years ago. Every day when you wake up, you can't simply go to the fridge and get something to eat. You must earn your food for the day by hunting for it.

Therefore, a lot of hunters had to fast because there wasn't anything to eat in the morning. Fast-forward to the present day and things are much different. Today, there's an overabundance of food. Anytime you want, you can drive through a 24/7 fast food restaurant and get something to eat.

You don't have to burn calories hunting for your food; you get in your car and drive to go get it. This is part of the reason why there is an obesity epidemic in America. Yes, having convenient restaurants and grocery stores is awesome, but they come at a price.

We're no longer forced to delay eating or have to earn it with exercise. How many people tell themselves, "I'll only eat this burger if I exercise for 30 minutes," or, "I'll eat this burger for lunch, but I won't eat anything else until then so I don't overeat." No one does this! It's easier to eat the burger now and worry about the consequences later.

Are We Even Meant to Eat Breakfast Anyway?

You've undoubtedly heard things before like, "Breakfast is the most important meal of the day," or, "Start your day off right with a good balanced breakfast." But were we even meant to eat breakfast anyway? Our ancestors didn't eat breakfast.

They had to wake up and hunt for their food. They didn't have an endless amount of cereal and pastries at their fingertips right when they woke up. So what happened? It wasn't until the 15th century that the word breakfast came into use in written English to describe a morning meal. So the idea of breakfast has been around for quite some time, but it wasn't until recently that it became popularized. It all started with two men, Will Keith Kellogg and C.W. Post, creating their own cereal companies—Kellogg Company and Postum Cereal Company (now known as Post Cereals). The key to these companies' success came down to two factors—sugar and marketing.

Thanks to a barrage of advertising, cereal was able to maintain a reputation that it was a healthy food. It would even go as far as to claim that cereal cured everything up to malaria and appendicitis. This was even the start of claims such as, "a good source of Vitamin D!"

And to appeal to children, companies created cartoon mascots such as Tony the Tiger and Snap, Crackle, and Pop, which started appearing around the 1930s. Finally, there's the phrase, "breakfast is the most important meal of the day." Cereal companies must first convince you to eat breakfast, and then get you to buy their cereal.

If they can do that, then they're in the clear because most people eat the same thing for breakfast everyday. Additionally, cereal was fast and convenient to make, which became increasingly important as corporate America was developing in the industrial age. Breakfast is a meal just like lunch or dinner. And while it may not be the most important, it certainly is the most marketed meal of the three.

Chapter 4: Benefits of Fasting

Aside from making fat loss a breeze, what else can you expect to gain from fasting? Quite a few things as it turns out...

-Live a longer life: There is evidence to suggest that fasting can help improve lifespan (3).

-Your body will become more efficient at using fat for fuel (4): When you fast, your body becomes glycogen depleted. Your body will then use fat stores for energy, and therefore learn to use fat for fuel for more effectively.

-Fasting can help to improve cognitive brain function, which will help to improve learning (5).

-Increased human growth hormone levels (hgh) (6): HGH is an important hormone for developing a lean and muscular body. It's responsible for muscle and bone growth, regulation of fluids, and regulation of body composition.

-You'll save time and money: Think about it. You won't have to spend as much time preparing, cooking, and eating meals. Plus, you'll save money at the grocery store!

-Improve focus and concentration: Have you ever felt sluggish or sleepy after eating a meal? The reason is because carbs make tryptophan more accessible to the brain. The tryptophan gets converted into serotonin, which eventually turns into melatonin. Melatonin regulates sleep and increases drowsiness. Therefore, by skipping breakfast you'll be more alert and focused, allowing you to be more productive in the morning.

-Faster recovery from sickness: There is evidence to suggest that fasting can help the body save energy and reduce heat loss, thus allowing it to focus solely on fighting off infection (7).

-Fasting may have positive effects on insulin resistance, thus reducing risk for type 2 diabetes (8).

-Fasting can help to reduce total cholesterol, blood pressure, and triglycerides (9).

Chapter 5: Different Methods of Fasting

Now it's time for the fun part. How exactly do you fast? Do you fast as long as you want and call it a day? Should you fast all day?

How often should you fast? As it turns out, there are quite a few different styles of fasting that exist. I'll share with you the pros and cons of each, and I'll tell you which method is best for long-term sustainability.

Fasting Method #1: The Warrior Diet

Ori Hofmekler created this style of fasting, and it involves a monstrous 20-hour daily fast and a 4-hour feeding window. This is definitely on the extreme end considering you'll be fasting for about 83% of the time in a day. You'll eat small amounts of fruits and vegetables during the day.

Then at night you'll get to enjoy a large feast. You can eat to your heart's content during your meal. It's unlikely that you'll overeat your allotted calories during one meal.

Typical number of meals per day: 1

Pros of the Warrior Diet:

-Easy way to ensure fat loss because it's unlikely you'll overeat from 1 meal.
-You'll get to enjoy a large amount of calories in 1 meal.
-You can enjoy eating your favorite foods with little worry of overeating.

Cons of the Warrior Diet:

-Its tough. Fasting for 20 hours a day can be hard to get used to.

-Not a flexible diet. Imagine your coworkers want you to come grab lunch with them. You can't go. Or maybe there's a birthday party you go to one weekend afternoon. You can't eat at the party. All of your social events must revolve around that 4-hour feeding window. Since that period of time is so small, it's unlikely to happen. You'll be forced to either cheat on your nutrition plan, or be "that guy" who's too good to eat at a party.

Fasting Method #2: Eat Stop Eat

Brad Pilon is the inventor of this style of fasting, and it involves doing a 24-hour fast 1-2 times per week. The main goal with this is to reduce your total caloric intake by 10-15% through fasting. The rest of the time you'll eat as you normally would.

For example, let's say you're going to do a 24-hour fast on a Wednesday and you start the fast at noon. You won't be able to eat anything until noon on Thursday. The key is to sleep during the hardest part of the fast. So if you notice you get really hungry after fasting for 12 hours, time it to where you go to sleep around the 12-hour mark.

Typical number of meals per day: 3

Pros of Eat Stop Eat:

-Easy way to control calories once you adapt to it.
-This method allows you to eat as you normally would when you're not fasting.
-Flexible enough to allow you to choose when you want to start the fast.
-You can sleep during the hardest part of the fast.

Cons of Eat Stop Eat:

-Can be hard to adapt to since you're only fasting 1-2 days per week and the fast is for 24 hours.

-Can be intrusive to your life on days that you fast. For example, you can't eat with friends or family on days you fast and working around this often can be tough.

Fasting Method #3: The 5:2 Diet

This method of fasting is similar to Eat Stop Eat. Popularized by Michael Mosley, this nutrition plan involves eating as you normally would 5 days of the week and only eating 500-600 calories on the other 2 days. For example, you would eat as you normally would every day except for Tuesday and Friday. On these days you would eat two small meals of around 250 calories each for women and 300 for men.

Typical number of meals per day: 3 on non-fasting days, 2 on fasting days

Pros of the 5:2 Diet:

-This plan allows you to start losing weight without changing any of the foods you typically eat.
-You get to eat two small meals on fasting days whenever you want. This provides you with *some* flexibility to eat with friends and family.
-You'll be eating the way you normally do the majority of the time.

Cons of The 5:2 Diet

-You fast infrequently (only two days per week) making it hard to adapt to.
-There's a drastic difference between days when you fast and days you don't fast, making it hard to get used to.
-It's possible to be social and eat with friends on fasting days, but the possibility of overeating during these meals is high.

Fasting Method #4: Fasting Every Other Day

This is an extreme method of fasting that involves fasting every other day. You'll eat as you normally would one day, and then fast the next day. There are different variations to this style of fasting that allow you to eat 500 calories on your fasting days. If you can pull it off, you'll definitely see some results; it's unlikely you'll overeat from only consuming calories 3-4 days per week.

Typical number of meals per day: 3 on non-fasting days, 0 on fasting days

Pros of Fasting Every Other Day

-Very likely to see weight loss results.
-You can eat as you normally would during non-fasting days.

Cons of Fasting Every Other Day

-Not for beginners. Don't try if you've never done fasting before.
-Too extreme for most people to handle.
-Frequent fasting makes it difficult to enjoy social meals with friends and family.
-Not necessary to start seeing results.

Fasting Method #5: The Leangains Method

Mark Berkhan popularized this style of fasting and it involves a daily fast of 16 hours and a feeding window of 8 hours. Typically, you'll eat 3 meals every 4 hours. For example, let's say your last meal of the day was at 8 p.m. You would fast until noon the next day and have meals at the following times:

Meal #1: Noon
Meal #2: 4:00 p.m.
Meal #3: 8:00 p.m.

Essentially what this boils down to is skipping breakfast. Yes, it'll take some time to adapt to this style of eating, but it fits in seamlessly with most lifestyles.

Typical number of meals per day: 3

Pros of Leansgains:

-Daily fasting makes it easy to stick to once you get used to it.
-You're only skipping breakfast, which isn't a meal you typically eat with friends anyway.
-You still get to consume 3 meals a day.
-Fairly effortless and easy way to control calories.

Cons of Leangains
-More flexibility than most fasting methods, but it could still do better. For example, what do you do if you stay up late one night until 2 a.m.? You wouldn't be allowed to eat anything past 8 p.m. using the schedule from above. Wouldn't it be better if you could eat at 2 a.m. and start your next fast from there?

Fasting Method #6: Flex Fasting

Who popularized flex fasting? No one. It's a name I made up for this style of fasting because it sounds cool. Flex fasting is a modified version of the Leangains method of fasting.

Instead of having a strict 16-hour fast and 8 hour feeding window, you'll simply push your first meal of the day back 4-5 hours after you wake up. It doesn't matter when your last meal of the day is, or what time you go to bed at. All you need to do is follow one simple rule—wake up and don't eat for at least 4-5 hours. For example, if you wake up at 8:00 a.m., don't eat anything until noon or 1:00 p.m.

Sometimes you'll only end up fasting for 12 hours, and other times you'll fast for up to 18 hours. Generally, you'll hover around the 14-16 hour mark and that's great. The main idea isn't to have some strict amount of time you have to fast for. The key is to have flexibility.

This way you can enjoy life *while* you lose weight. You're in control of your diet, and your diet no longer calls the shots. Think about it. Most diets give you specific times and boring foods you must eat at those times.

It doesn't matter if you're hungry, or if you're in the mood to eat those foods. You must do it to lose weight. Your life must revolve around fitness in order for it to work. Most people realize it isn't worth it (because it's definitely not) and they quit.

Fortunately, flex fasting gives you a better option. Yes, I'm biased towards this fasting method, but remember, *all* of the fasting methods outlined here will work. You have to pick which one you think will work best for you and try it out. You'll never know until you give it a shot.

I've personally been doing fasting for about 4 years now and I've tried many different methods. During my first two years of fasting, I flip flopped between many of the different styles, and I never found one that was a homerun for me. Then I started doing flex fasting, and it has by far been the easiest method for me to stick with. It fits in seamlessly with my life.

I don't get crazy hungry because I have to fast 20 hours a day or anything like that. It has the best balance between structure and flexibility, which is why I recommend trying it for yourself.

Typical number of meals per day: 3

Pros of Flex Fasting:

-Extremely flexible for most schedules.
-Easy and effortless way to control calories.

-Will allow you to still be able to eat social meals with friends.

Cons of Flex Fasting:

-Lacks rigid structure. This makes it easy to bend the rules or not follow them at all.

Fasting Method #7: Skip Meals When Convenient

This last method isn't a structured fasting protocol like the previous ones are. It simply involves you skipping meals when it's convenient to do so or when you're not hungry. This gives you maximum flexibility, but the complete lack of structure will make it difficult to obtain any lasting results.

How often do we get around to doing something when it's convenient? Hardly ever because when it's not convenient to do something, we'll delay taking action.

Typical number of meals per day: 1-3

Pros of Skipping Meals When Convenient

-Provides maximum flexibility allowing for seamless fit into any lifestyle or schedule.
-Easy nutrition plan to get started with—simply start skipping meals when you can.

Cons of Skipping Meals When Convenient

-Lacks structure making it easy to not take any action.
-Unlikely to provide any results because you're only skipping meals when you feel like it, which will be few and far between.
Pick One and Get Started
Now that you know the different methods of fasting the main thing is to get started. Choose the style you think will work best for you and try it out. If you're not sure which one to

pick, start with method #6—flex fasting. Be sure to test it out for 2 weeks before moving on to a different method. Don't let all of the different choices paralyze you into not taking action. If you've never done fasting before you won't know what works best for you until you start testing the choices out.

Chapter 6: Fasting and Exercise

Not only can you use fasting as a great nutrition strategy, but you can also use it to help maximize fat loss in the gym. There are a couple of different ways to take advantage of this. The first way is by being in a fasted state when you workout. All you need to do is workout in the morning or early afternoon before you've eaten anything.

When you workout in a fed state, your body will use the glycogen in your body as fuel for energy. However when you workout fasted, your body will be glycogen depleted. This means that your body won't be able to tap into your glycogen stores for energy, it'll have to go somewhere else. Guess where that somewhere else is? Your fat stores!

So by working out in a fasted state, your body will become more efficient at using fat for energy instead of carbs. The second thing you can do to maximize fat loss from working out is delay eating after your workout. The media has done a good job of making us think we must immediately consume protein after a workout or else it was a waste. Research shows that your body won't lose muscle if you don't eat protein within 45 minutes of your workout (10).

Whenever you workout, your body's growth hormone levels will increase (11). This growth hormone will help to protect your muscle and increase fat burning. However if you eat right after you finish a workout, your growth hormone levels will be blunted and insulin levels will increase. For this reason, you'll want to delay eating anything after finishing a workout for 1-2 hours.

Eating more calories won't help you lose more weight. Yet when it comes to eating after a workout, people act like they're immune to gaining fat from these extra calories. "I hit it hard in the gym today, I deserve a large milkshake!" No, you don't.

Imagine you go to the gym and burn 300 calories. Then, immediately after your workout, you consume a 350-calorie post workout protein shake. Now you've completely wiped out all of the calories you burned from the workout, plus you ate an additional 50 calories! It's ok to eat a meal after working out if that's when you would normally eat anyway.

Don't go out of your way to eat extra calories for the sake of a post workout shake—it won't help you burn more fat! You might be weary of working out fasted if you usually workout in a fed state. Give it a try for 1-2 weeks to give your body a chance to adapt to it. Once you do, you should notice that you have more focus and intensity in the gym.

Here's a good beginner's workout plan you can do if you're unsure of what to do in the gym (a more advanced workout will be provided later on in the book):
This regimen consists of 3 full-body weight workouts per week. You'll complete the same workout every time you go to the gym. You can set up your workout schedule in one of the following ways:

Monday: Workout
Tuesday: Rest
Wednesday: Workout
Thursday: Rest
Friday: Workout
Saturday: Rest
Sunday: Rest

Or

Monday: Rest
Tuesday: Workout
Wednesday: Rest
Thursday: Rest
Friday: Rest
Saturday: Rest
Sunday: Rest

As a beginner, full-body workouts will provide you with many benefits:

-You'll burn more calories from your workouts.
-You'll gain strength and muscle faster since you'll be stimulating your muscles more frequently.
-You'll have better nervous system recovery because you won't train on consecutive days.
-You'll develop perfect form on key lifts faster because you practice them more often.

Essentially your body has never been exposed to this stimulus (i.e. weightlifting) before. Therefore, you can take advantage of what some people call "newbie gains." And by increasing the frequency at which you stimulate your muscle groups, you can speed up the process.

Side Note: A set is a group of consecutive repetitions. A repetition is one complete motion of an exercise. And the rest period is how long of a break you'll take until you start the next set. For example, let's say you're completing 3 sets of 8 reps and resting 2 minutes in between sets for the barbell squat exercise.

You'll squat down and stand back up, completing the motion of the exercise and one rep. You'll repeat that motion 7 more times for a total of 8 repetitions. That will complete the set and you will begin your rest period. Once your 2-minute rest period is up, you'll start the next set and perform another 8 repetitions.

That will complete set number 2, and you'll rest another 2 minutes. Once that time period is up, you'll complete the final set of 8 repetitions, and then you'll move onto the next exercise.

Here's the workout:

- Incline Barbell Bench Press: 3 sets 8 reps 2 min rest between (btw) sets
- Barbell Back Squats: 3 sets of 8 reps 2 min rest btw sets
- Lat Pulldowns: 3 sets of 10 reps 90 sec rest btw sets
- Seated DB Military Press: 3 sets of 8 reps 2 min rest btw sets
- Standing DB Curls: 3 sets of 12 reps 60 sec rest btw sets
- Tricep Rope Pushdowns: 3 sets of 12 reps 60 sec rest btw sets

That's all there is to it! Don't let the simplicity of it fool you—it will work.

Chapter 7: Fasting and Building Muscle

When it comes to intermittent fasting, most people tend to think of fat loss. Believe it or not, intermittent fasting can also be an effective nutrition strategy for building muscle. Recall some of the benefits I mentioned earlier about fasting—specifically increased growth hormone and increased efficiency using fat for fuel.

The additional growth hormone will help you build more muscle, and you'll be less likely to store fat while you pack on muscle. So then what's the difference between fasting for fat loss and fasting to build muscle? The answer lies in the amount of calories you need to eat. The caloric deficit is king for fat loss, and the caloric surplus is king for building muscle.

This means you must eat more calories than you burn off if you want to build muscle. Imagine you're an architect building a 2,600 square foot house. You'll need a certain number of bricks—say 6,000 for example—in order to build that house. If you don't have 6,000 bricks, then you'll have to downgrade the size of the house you're building.

Your muscles work the same way. If you want to build muscle, you must provide your body with enough of the raw materials (i.e. calories you get from food) necessary for it to happen. If you don't, then you'll be in the same boat as an architect without enough bricks. How many calories do you need to build muscle?

Use this simple equation:

Bodyweight in pounds x16=Daily caloric intake
Using myself as an example:

Bodyweight-195x16=3,120 calories

This means that I need to eat 3,120 calories everyday in order to start gaining weight. One common complaint from guys is that they're a "hardgainer" or that they have a lightning fast metabolism. It doesn't matter how much they eat, they can't seem to gain any weight. The issue isn't that you're a hardgainer, it's the fact that you're not measuring how much you're eating.

You might *think* you eat a lot of calories, but until you actually track it how will you know? Simply put—you won't. The first thing you'll need to do is measure your weight. You have to know what your starting point is. From there, measure the number of calories in everything you eat and record it.

Use Google, My Fitness Pal, nutrition labels, and anything else you can to get an idea of how much you're eating. It'll never be exact, and that's ok. You want to get a rough measurement of how much you're eating. From there, track the calories in the note app on your phone.

For example, let's say this is what you ate one day:

Breakfast: Protein Shake
Lunch: Chicken Salad
Dinner: Hamburger and fries

You'd find out about how many calories were in each meal you ate and record it as follows:

2/5/17
Meal 1: 600 calories
Meal 2: 450 calories
Meal 3: 850 calories
Total calories for the day: 1,900

Bam, it's that simple! After doing this for a week, measure your weight again. If you didn't gain any weight, then add 200 calories to your total daily number and eat that much for the following week. In my case for example, I would add 200 to my original number of 3,120 and get 3,320 daily calories.

Keep repeating this process until you start gaining .5-1 pound per week. If you're gaining more than 1 pound per week, then you're likely gaining too much fat and you'll need to cut back. Yes, it can be hard to eat 3,000+ calories in a day, but that doesn't give you the excuse to consume high-calorie junk food all the time.

Eating 3,000 calories worth of chips, candy, and fries will not give you the same muscle building results as eating high quality foods like chicken breasts, brown rice, and vegetables. This isn't to say that you can never consume junk food, but the majority of your diet needs to consist of high-quality, wholesome foods. My rule is to eat clean foods about 85% of the time and fill in the remaining 15% with my favorite foods like chocolate chip ice cream, pizza, and potato chips.

If you can do that, you'll be golden. So what are some easy ways to consume enough high quality calories? Here are some suggestions:

#1 Make Monster Protein Shakes

Protein shakes are one of the easiest ways to consume more calories. It's far easier to drink your calories than eat them. Make the following shake and consume it in between meals or as a meal replacement when you're short on time:

1 Frozen Banana (105 calories)
¼ Cup Frozen Blueberries (21 calories)
1 Tablespoon Olive Oil (120 calories)
1 Cup of Oatmeal (300 calories)
2 Scoops of Protein Powder (240 calories)
1-2 Cups of Milk (100-200 calories)
Total Calories: 886-986

#2 Consume More High Quality Fats

Fat has gotten a bad name over the years. People think if they eat fat, then they will gain fat. Not true! Fat helps with digestion, insulation, and nervous system function (12).

Not only that, but it's a great way to consume more calories if you want to build muscle! Fat contains 9 calories per gram opposed to protein and carbs, which only contain 4 calories per gram. So you're getting twice the amount of calories per gram when you consume fat! Obviously though, you want to consume high quality fats like mono and polyunsaturated fats instead of getting fat from French fries and chips.

Here's a list of high quality fats you can eat to hit your daily caloric intake:

- Coconut oil
- Olive oil
- Flaxseed oil
- Cashews
- Walnuts
- Peanuts
- Natural Peanut Butter
- Natural Almond Butter

#3 Eat More Foods that are Easy to Consume

Consuming more foods like Greek yogurt, mashed potatoes, and cottage cheese is another great way to squeeze in more calories. These foods don't require you to chew a lot, making it easier for you consume them like the protein shake. As far as Greek yogurt is concerned, buy it in a big container. Then add 1-2 scoops of your favorite protein powder to it with blueberries or raspberries for a tasty snack.

You'll want to get the plain version of Greek yogurt because flavored yogurt (like vanilla or strawberry) will have too much added sugar in it. Normally the plain version will taste bland, but it won't if you add in the protein powder and fruit. Mashed potatoes are another great source of carbs. I like eating them with a source of lean meat and vegetables for a complete meal.

Finally, cottage cheese is also a great food to snack on. It's high in protein and low in fat. Not only that, but it's a casein protein, which means it's slower digesting. This makes cottage cheese a great food to eat before bedtime to give you a constant release of protein throughout the night!

#4: Protein Bars

Protein bars are another great way to get some extra calories (and protein) in, no matter where you're at. If you're on a quick break at work, or you're away from home, a protein bar is a quick and simple snack. Of course quality is key here. Many protein bars on the market are garbage and will only provide you with simple sugars and preservatives.

My favorites are Quest and Oh Yeah! They're a little bit more expensive, but worth the extra price. Remember, you get what you pay for! The largest downside to protein bars is the price. You're essentially paying for the convenience of having packaged ready-eat-to protein. If you're on a budget, don't sweat it, you still have plenty of other ways to consume more calories.

Setting Up Your Macronutrients

A macronutrient is a type of food that is required in large amounts in the human diet. There are 3 macronutrients—protein, carbs, and fat. All 3 macronutrients are important regardless of what your fitness goals are. This is how much of each macronutrient you should eat:

40% of your total calories from protein
40% of your total calories from carbs
20% of your total calories from fat

This is how you would calculate actual numbers for each macronutrient, using myself as an example:

Bodyweight (195) x16= 3,120 calories
.4x 3,120=1,248 daily calories from protein
.4x 3,120=1,248 daily calories from carbs
.2x 3,120=624 daily calories from fat

At first glance, this might seem like you're eating too many carbs. Carbs are crucial for the muscle building process, and they'll help provide you with plenty of energy to crush it during your workouts. You won't gain fat from carbs unless you're eating too many calories overall.

As long as you're in that sweet spot where you're eating enough to build muscle, but not enough to gain excessive fat, you'll be good to go. Lastly, don't worry about hitting these numbers spot on. Use them to help guide you. If you can stay within 5% of what I recommend, you'll be well on your way to packing on muscle.

Chapter 8: Muscle Building Workout With Fasting

Nutrition is only half the battle when it comes to building muscle. You must workout as well. Your training is what will provide your body with a stimulus telling it to grow bigger and stronger to handle the stress it underwent.

What's more important for building the ultimate physique—nutrition or training? That's similar to asking what's more important for your survival—food or water? You need both food and water to survive, and you need both proper nutrition and training to build your best body.

Follow this workout to build muscle:

This workout contains 4 workouts per week. It contains 2 different workouts—A and B. You'll alternate between workout A and B every time you go to the gym. Set up your gym schedule in 1 of the following 2 ways:

Monday: Workout A
Tuesday: Workout B
Wednesday: Rest Day
Thursday: Workout A
Friday: Workout B
Saturday: Rest Day
Sunday: Rest Day

Or

Monday: Workout A
Tuesday: Workout B
Wednesday: Rest Day
Thursday: Workout A
Friday: Rest Day
Saturday: Workout B
Sunday: Off

The second option will give you an extra day of rest in between workouts, which will help with central nervous system recovery. Feel free to pick whatever best fits your schedule.

Workout A: Chest, Shoulders, and Triceps

- Incline Barbell or Dumbbell Bench Press: 3 sets of 6 reps 3 min rest btw sets
- Seated Dumbbell Military Press: 3 sets of 6 reps 3 min rest btw sets
- Dumbbell Skull Crushers: 3 sets of 8 reps 90 sec rest btw sets
- Standing Dumbbell Lateral Raises: 3 sets of 10-12 reps 60 sec rest btw sets
- Bent Lateral Raises: 3 sets of 10-12 reps 60 sec rest btw sets

Workout B: Back, Biceps, and Legs

- Weighted Pull-Ups (replace with lat pulldowns if you're unable to do pull-ups): 3 sets of 6 reps 3 min rest btw sets
- Incline Dumbbell Curls: 3 sets of 8 reps 90 sec rest btw sets
- Bulgarian Split Squats: 3 sets of 8 reps (per leg) 2 min rest btw sets
- Bent Over Row: 3 sets of 8 reps 2 min rest btw sets
- Hammer Curls: 3 sets of 10-12 reps 60 sec rest btw sets

Chapter 9: How You Can Actually Be Successful With Your Fitness Journey

This book has provided you with the tools that you need to be successful with fitness. However, simply having the tools isn't always enough. Your mindset is also an essential component. Some people fail because they're using the wrong tools (i.e. restrictive diets or insane workouts), but many others fail before the journey has even begun due to their mentality.

People think that once they get a killer body, their lives will magically change. Women will be all over them, their relationships will improve, they'll get a raise at work, or whatever else. Few if any of those things will actually happen once you get in shape. Yes, you'll get compliments along the way from your friends and family, which will feel good, but don't expect to have your choice of super models to date.

The real prize that comes from getting into shape is the person you'll become. It takes a lot of discipline, self-motivation, and persistence to get in great shape. These are the qualities you'll be developing in yourself on your fitness journey. Once you do reach your fitness goal, you'll not only have these characteristics deeply ingrained inside of you, but you'll also have the body of your dreams.

The self-growth and self-improvement will be the core reason why someone would become more attracted to you, or why you would get a raise at work. My senior year of high school, I scored 28 points during the opening game of the basketball season. It was an incredible feeling that I'll never forget. But what made that moment so special?

I felt ecstatic because I earned it. Nobody gave me those 28 points—I had worked hard for them by developing my skills during the offseason. I was putting in the work alone in the gym when nobody else was watching. It was never about showing off or looking cool in front of other people.

In fact, it wasn't even about trying to put up huge numbers during games. It was about doing what I loved. I loved basketball, whether I was playing in a competitive game or shooting in my backyard. I was after the process, not the prize; that's why I succeeded.

I carried this same philosophy into my fitness training, and it's how you'll be successful with it as well. Of course, this sounds counter-intuitive. But look around and you'll notice that most people *only* want the prize and want nothing to do with the process. That's why they fail.

Take lottery winners for example. Wouldn't it be cool to win millions of dollars? Studies show otherwise (13). Roughly 44% of lottery winners lose all of their earnings within 5 years.
They go through divorce, drug abuse, robberies, and other tragedies. Their so-called "friends" and family will start to hound them for money. The same thing would happen if there was a weight loss pill that would have you waking up with a six-pack. You wouldn't learn anything from it, and you'd quickly gain the weight back.

You must accept where you're at right now. Everyone has to start from somewhere, and it'll only get better from here. Beyond that, you must find a way to make the process enjoyable. This is the only way you'll go to the gym and stick to a nutrition plan for a long time to come.

Not banning your favorite foods is the best and easiest way to make dieting more enjoyable. Finally, understand that fitness is a lifelong journey and not a sprint. This will take a lot of the pressure off you to feel like you have to succeed tomorrow.

Take a step back. Breathe. And *always* stay true to the process. That's how you'll flourish.

Chapter 10: Frequently Asked Questions

How much weight should I lift during the workouts?

Lift as much weight as you possibly can for the given rep range. Initially, you won't know how much weight to use so you'll have to take your best guess. For example, let's say you're doing bench press for 8 reps. You think you can lift around 150 pounds for that many reps, but on your first set you easily complete 10 reps.

This means the weight is too light and you need to increase it for the next set. On the next set you lift 165 pounds and struggle to complete the 8th rep. This is what you want to happen and it means you've found a good weight to use. Once you can complete all 3 sets for 8 reps with 165 pounds, move up to 170 the next time you bench press. If you can't complete 8 reps for all 3 sets stick with 165 until you can. Here's an example:

Workout 1: Bench Press with 165 pounds
Set 1: 8 reps
Set 2: 8 reps
Set 3: 7 reps

Because you only completed 7 reps on the last set, stick with 165 for the next workout—

Workout 2: Bench Press with 165 pounds
Set 1: 8 reps
Set 2: 8 reps
Set 3: 8 reps

Because you completed all 3 sets for 8 reps move up to 170 on your next workout with bench press.

Note: It's better to use a weight that's too heavy and miss a rep or two than it is to use a weight that's too light and leave some reps in the tank. For example, it's better to do 170 pounds and only complete 6 reps instead of 8 opposed to using 155 pounds and stopping at 8 reps even though you could've easily done more reps.

Should I Do Cardio?

Doing cardio depends on what your fitness goals are. If you're looking to build muscle, then pass on cardio aside from doing some walking here and there. If you're looking to burn fat, than cardio can definitely be a handy tool to help you out. Cardio will do one of two things for you:

#1: Speed up the rate at which you lose fat.
Or

#2: Give you some extra leeway in your diet.

Cardio is by no means necessary for you to reach your fat loss goals, but it will help. What type of cardio should you do—slow and steady or running? Science shows that the best type of cardio you can do is something called high intensity interval training (HIIT) (14).

This kind of cardio combines high intensity cardio with low intensity cardio. HIIT by itself is very effective, but it can be maximized when you immediately follow it with slow steady state cardio. The intensity of the HIIT will release free fatty acids into your bloodstream, and the slow steady state cardio will burn them off. Here's how to perform this hybrid cardio workout:

Part 1: HIIT

Alternate between a high intensity and a low intensity for 10-15 minutes on your choice of cardio machine. Here's an example on a treadmill:
-Run at 7.5 mph for 1 minute

-Walk at 3.5 mph for 1 minute
-Repeat for 10-15 minutes

Part 2: Slow steady state cardio (done immediately after HIIT)

Example on a treadmill: Walk at a constant pace of 3.5-4 mph for 10-15 minutes

Note: If you need to adjust the intensity of the HIIT then do so. You can alter the run-walk ratios (i.e. run for 30 seconds and walk for 1.5 minutes), or you can decrease the intensity of each run (i.e. run at 6 mph instead of 7.5). And if what I prescribed is too easy, then ramp up the intensity accordingly.

How Fast Should I Lose Weight?

The more weight you have to lose, the faster the rate at which you can lose the weight. For example, if you have 50+ pounds to lose, you can lose weight at a rate of 2 pounds or more per week. If you only have 5 pounds to lose, then lose weight at a rate of .5 pound per week.

For most people, losing 1 pound per week is the sweet spot. You'll be creating an average caloric deficit of 500 calories daily. At this pace, you'll be losing weight fairly quickly and you won't be miserable all of the time from a complete lack of calories.

What Am I Allowed to Drink During a Fast?

The only drinks you're allowed to have during a fast are drinks that contain zero to a few calories (10 or less). Drinking something like a soda or orange juice would break the fast and stop all of the benefits from the fast. Here's a list of acceptable drinks you can have during a fast:

- Water

- Green Tea
- Black Coffee
- Diet Soda
- Water Flavorings that Don't Contain any Calories

What Should I Eat When I'm Not Fasting?

This is a tricky question to answer, and it relates to that old phrase, "If you give a man a fish, you feed him for a day, but if you teach him how to fish you feed him for life." If I tell you what to eat for every meal, than I am giving you a fish.

You're not going to learn anything. You won't know how to adapt and eat if you're away from home for example. But if I teach you *how* to eat, then I can teach you how to stay lean for the rest of your life. I'll give you some guidelines to follow, but don't feel the need to stick with them 100% of the time:

Guideline #1: Above all else—burn off more calories than you consume.

Nothing else matters if you're not in a caloric deficit. Many people seem to forget about this and think if they eat healthy, then they're guaranteed to lose weight. Yes, healthy foods are *generally* lower in calories than unhealthy foods, but eating healthy doesn't guarantee anything. Being in a caloric deficit will guarantee weight loss.

Guideline #2: Eat wholesome, healthy foods roughly 85% of the time

Like I mentioned above, eating healthy isn't the only thing you need to lose weight, but it's still important. Not only do wholesome foods have fewer calories, but they're also more filling. Since your calories are going to be restricted, it's crucial that you make good use of the calories you do have.

For example, if you need to eat 1,700 calories a day to lose weight, using 1,000 of those calories to eat a burger and fries might not be the wisest decision. The following is a list of some high quality foods you should eat in your diet. This isn't a comprehensive list:

- Sweet potatoes
- Vegetables
- Fruit
- Lean Meats
- Nuts
- Cottage Cheese
- Oatmeal
- Brown Rice
- Quinoa
- Fish

You can fill in the remaining 15% of your diet with foods you enjoy. Eating your favorite foods is essential for fat loss as well, so don't skip on this! Leaning down can be a hard process, and eating your favorite foods will help keep you sane and make the journey far more enjoyable.

You know you're not going to go the rest of your life without eating ice cream or potato chips, so make room for them in your nutrition plan and enjoy it! Here's a list of some of my favorite foods:

- Mint chocolate chip ice cream
- Pizza
- Hamburgers
- Potato chips
- Popcorn
- Cookies
- Milkshakes

Guideline #3: Forgive yourself

Understand there will be times when you slip up and that's ok. What's not ok is to make the situation worse by saying, "screw it," and binge eating everything in sight. Give yourself permission to be human and make mistakes. Don't strive to be perfect 100% of the time, aim for 85%, and even when you don't reach 85%, forgive yourself.

Back when I was 16 and I first started working out, I would feel incredibly guilty if I even thought about eating a cookie. I would take pride in myself because I could resist temptation while others couldn't. But fitness felt like a chore, and I wasn't having fun with it. Don't be perfect—be the human that you are!

Guideline #4: Fill up on the healthy stuff first

Sometimes I'll be hungry for ice cream, but I'll tell myself I can only eat after I finish the rest of my meal. At times, I won't even end up eating any ice cream because I wasn't hungry for it after the main course. Even if I was, I wouldn't eat as much as I normally do because I filled up on the good stuff first. Whenever a craving hits you hard, do the same.

Foods that are high in protein like chicken breast and steak work great for this. These foods require a lot of chewing before you can swallow them, which will slow you down. High protein foods are also very satiating, so you might get full before you satisfy your sweet tooth.

Guideline #5: Know yourself and spread out your calories accordingly

Let's say for example you determine you need to eat 1,800 calories daily to lose weight. You'll do intermittent fasting for the first part of the day, and then eat 3 meals usually around 1:00, 5:00, and 9:00. You could bust up your allotted calories evenly, and eat 600 calories for each of your 3 meals, but you certainly don't have to.

For example, let's say you like to eat bigger meals later in the day before you go to bed. You could eat less calories during your first 2 meals and save the extra calories for your last meal when you would actually want to eat them. For instance:

Meal 1: 400 calories
Meal 2: 400 calories
Meal 3: 1,000 calories

Change this up based on however it is you like to eat. If you like eating more of your calories earlier in the day, then do so, but eat less at night. You don't have to evenly distribute your calories across meals if you don't want to.

Is there anything in particular I should eat to break my fast with?

No. Once you've completed your fast for the day, eat whatever meal you'd normally eat. It's kind of like coming back from the dentist after a teeth cleaning. You don't want to ruin that sparkly clean feeling, but something has to end it and fasting is no different. You can eat healthy or unhealthy to break a fast—either way is fine as long as you're still creating a caloric deficit!

How much water should I drink on a daily basis?

Your body is made up of about 60% water, so it's important to consume water for several reasons:

- It'll help keep your joints and ligaments fluid, which can help prevent injury.
- Water can help control your caloric intake.
- Flush out toxins
- Improve skin quality
- Improve kidney function
- Improve your focus
-

Many people recommend that you should drink 1 gallon of water per day. This is a blanket answer that doesn't meet individual needs. This recommendation would have a 100-pound woman drinking the same amount of water as a 200-pound man. Absurd!

Other health experts advise drinking eight 8-ounce glasses (64 ounces total) of water a day. But again 64 ounces isn't going to be enough for most people. What should you do then? I don't keep track of my water intake—I go by how I feel and the color of my urine.

Your body's own thirst mechanism will be accurate in telling you if you need more water. If you feel thirsty, then go drink some water. If not, then you're probably ok. You can also use the color of your urine to judge how hydrated you are. If your urine is yellow, then you should drink more water. If it's clear then you should be good to go. This keeps things simple and it's one less thing you have to keep track of.

How Do I Motivate Myself to Go to the Gym?

Finding the motivation to go to the gym or eat right can be hard. No matter who you are, there will be times when you don't feel like working out. Having that feeling is ok, but you can't let it control you. There will be times when you'll have to do it anyway even when you don't feel like it.

That's what will ultimately separate a long-term successful fitness journey from failing at it. I do have some tips to help you out along the way however:

Tip #1: Focus on Gradual Improvements

Many people make fitness an all-or-nothing game. They tell themselves that they'll workout 5 days a week and eat clean 100% of the time for the rest of their lives. Let's say you workout only 4 days one week. Are you a failure?

Of course not. You still worked out 4 days, but in your mind you are because you failed to reach 5 workouts. You make it hard to celebrate any small successes that you do have because the standards are too high.

Instead, focus on making smaller, more gradual improvements, and celebrate any successes you have along the way. For example, start off with a goal to only workout 2 days per week if it's been years since you've last worked out. Once you achieve that goal, you'll feel good about yourself, and you can move up to working out 3 days per week and so on.

Tip #2: Action Leads Motivation

People think they have to get the inspiration or motivation from somewhere in order to take the action necessary to workout. The reverse of that is actually true. You need to start by taking an action no matter how small. And once you get started you'll likely want to continue on with what you're doing.

When I think about everything I have to do to workout: put my gym clothes on, drive to the gym, workout with a bunch of grueling exercises, drive back, and shower—I start to make up silly excuses as to why I should skip this time. Instead I'll tell myself to do just one exercise when I get to the gym and not pressure myself to do anything more. After I finish that first exercise, it's always easier for me to finish the rest of the workout.

You just have to get started. Try this out for any healthy habit you want to start. For example, if you want to start flossing your teeth, tell yourself you'll only floss one tooth and don't pressure yourself to do anything more than that!

Tip #3: Put Your Own Money on the Line

Money is a very powerful motivator. And you can use your own money to motivate yourself to start working out more. Here's what you're going to do—give someone a good amount of money. Not $20, but something that would actually hurt you—$100, $200, $500, or whatever you can't afford to lose.

Then tell your friend that if you don't go to the gym 3 days this week for example, they get to keep the money. When you give up the money in the first place, you'll fight to get it back. This is much different than telling yourself you'll give the money to someone after you miss your workouts.

It's too easy to make an excuse and not give away the money. Give the money up in the first place and make sure your friend actually holds you accountable to it. This is by far the best way to get motivation to workout. There's a real cost involved if you don't comply. You'll either get ripped or go broke trying.

Sources

(1) https://www.bmc.org/nutrition-and-weight-management/weight-management

(2)https://www.ncbi.nlm.nih.gov/pubmed/22825659

(3)http://fitness.mercola.com/sites/fitness/archive/2016/03/25/health-benefits-fasting.aspx#_edn1

(4) https://www.ncbi.nlm.nih.gov/pubmed/371355

(5)https://www.ncbi.nlm.nih.gov/pmc/articles/PMC3289210/

(6)https://www.ncbi.nlm.nih.gov/pmc/articles/PMC329619/

(7)https://www.ncbi.nlm.nih.gov/pmc/articles/PMC4257368/

(8)https://www.ncbi.nlm.nih.gov/pubmed/24993615

(9)https://www.ncbi.nlm.nih.gov/pubmed/17929537

(10)https://www.ncbi.nlm.nih.gov/pubmed/22460474

(11)https://www.ncbi.nlm.nih.gov/pubmed/2796409

(12) https://www.ncbi.nlm.nih.gov/pubmed/15052493

(13) http://fortune.com/2016/01/15/powerball-lottery-winners/

(14) https://www.ncbi.nlm.nih.gov/pubmed/8028502

Printed in Great Britain
by Amazon